THE
Undiet Diet

THE
Undiet Diet

DEVELOP AND ACHIEVE GOOD HEALTH, WELL-BEING AND PERMANENT WEIGHT LOSS

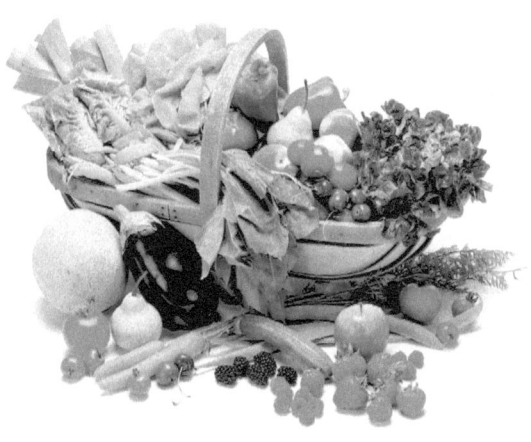

ANN GREENE

iUniverse, Inc.
Bloomington

The Undiet Diet
Develop and Achieve Good Health, Well-Being and Permanent Weight Loss

iUniverse books may be ordered through booksellers or by contacting:

iUniverse
1663 Liberty Drive
Bloomington, IN 47403
www.iuniverse.com
1-800-Authors (1-800-288-4677)

ISBN: 978-1-4697-9556-0 (sc)
ISBN: 978-1-4697-9557-7 (ebk)

Printed in the United States of America

If you are interested in submitting your success story in the next edition of the Undiet Diet, email: jayounglmt@yahoo.com

iUniverse rev. date: 03/23/2012

CONTENTS

To my husband and son who inspired and encouraged me to write this book. And a special thank you to my now deceased father, Bruce who helped with the original printing and artwork.

Also, to all those who are fighting a constant battle with trying to lose and maintain your desired weight.

INTRODUCTION

Whether you want to lose five or 350 pounds, these next pages should prove enlightening as well as inspiring.

This book is written from a perspective of personal experience with weight loss and improved health that has lasted for approximately seven years.

If you are interested and ready to commit yourself to a tested and proven, permanent weight loss program, then I invite you to read on. This is neither a fad diet nor a new exercise regime that will leave your entire body starved and burned out; it reveals how to successfully change your attitude and bad habits into a new desirable you.

The Undiet Diet is weight management. We will teach you how to incorporate healthy eating habits into your existing daily schedule. You will learn that your current eating and living habits may be the very culprits of excessive weight and poor health.

You will also learn secrets to transforming your body into a desirable shape that you will be proud to show off in public. Your energy level, as well as your self-esteem, will soar to new heights.

Are you ready to change your life for the better—forever? Let's get started.

Chapter 1

MY STORY

My husband, John and son, Sean and I had just relocated to central North Carolina, and I was lucky enough to find employment with one of the largest and the most profitable pharmaceutical companies in the world. John was happy in his line of work as a salesman, and Sean was content in his elementary school. Things looked great and we were off to a wonderful, new start in life.

As our second Christmas in North Carolina approached, I was looking forward to holiday vacation. We planned a trip to the mountains for winter sports and some sightseeing. Suddenly, I developed a fever. When I awoke the next day, my throat felt like raging flames of fire and my fever had spiked to 104°. John finally insisted I visit the doctor. After a few tests, it was determined that I had the flu and strep throat. The doctor prescribed strong antibiotics and advised I go home, rest and drink plenty of water. I did, and in about seven days felt well and renewed.

It wasn't until ten days after my last prescription pill was taken when I discovered a large, deep-rooted and welt-like pimple on my left leg. It was extremely painful to the touch.

I ignored it thinking I had an ingrown hair or clogged pores. After one week, the large pimple was still there, and I noticed another welt on the same leg closer to my ankle. Two more days later, another welt appeared, similar in size and also very painful. This concerned me greatly, so I visited the doctor. After an exam and my doctor consulting with two other physicians in the office, they concluded that I might have an allergic reaction to the medication he prescribed for my prior strep throat. I was swiftly referred to a dermatologist in the Durham area. As the dermatologist examined the welts on my legs, which now had spread to both legs from my ankles to my upper thighs, she called in another doctor to ask for his opinion. After a series of tests and another appointment, it was determined that I had erythema nodosum, which was described to me as a reaction from strep. The doctor's medical instructions to me were to stay out of work for about one month, take 4 Motrin pills 4 times a day and keep my legs elevated. No other medication was prescribed. John and I were outraged at what we considered poor medical advice. Two more weeks passed, and the erythema nodosum spread like wild fire on a dry, windy day. I decided to get a second opinion from another dermatologist. Once again I had to get another referral from my primary care doctor, and with much stress and aggravation, I obtained an appointment with someone in Raleigh, North Carolina. Since this is a rare disease with few known cases, when the second dermatologist called in her associate to look at my legs, both unanimously agreed that it was erythema nodosum, a side effect from strep throat. She prescribed ampicillin and a prescription five times stronger than Motrin. In two months, I felt better and saw a great improvement. It took four long and agonizing months for the erythema nodosum to disappear. It took an additional year for the scars to completely fade.

During my illness, I began reading everything I could get my hands on, including surfing the Internet for information about my illness and cures in both the conventional and alternative medical press. In talking with one of my co-workers, she referred me to a wonderful Iridologist who put me on natural remedies. I asked my husband, John for a Juiceman juicer for my birthday that year. I strongly believe that using my juicer, natural remedies and changing the way I ate, put me on the path to better health. During this period when I changed my way of eating and began juicing, is when I lost all my excess weight. To this day, I am maintaining a constant weight of 113 pounds. I am now 49 years old and have more energy, awareness and feel better than when I was in my 20's.

As my health improved, I made a promise to God and myself in dedicating my life to spreading the word about how to achieve good health. It is not the profit that is motivating me, but the feelings of accomplishment in helping others achieve what I have discovered—excellent health.

Chapter 2

WHY DO I OVER EAT?

No matter how much I cut back on my food consumption, from sacrificing ice cream to candy bars, I still weighed over 30 pounds more than I wanted to. I joined a health spa and visited faithfully three to four times a week, trying all the free weights, strength training weights, and joining high impact aerobics classes, but the scales still read, "tilt." I filled my freezer with all varieties of lean cuisine dinners that I found in the store, than ran straight to my health spa. After several months of this frustrating routine only to have lost one or two pounds, I became emotionally upset and gave up, reverting back to my destructive eating habits and lifestyle. Needless to say, I gained back my entire original weight plus five additional pounds. I was so depressed that I wallowed in self-pity, shut out the world, and ate constantly everyday until I fell asleep at night.

Does this scenario sound familiar? What went wrong here? First, I did not eat the *right* foods, therefore my workout could not have possibly burned off all the calories and fat I consumed. I also expected Polaroid results. In today's fast pace, we expect results yesterday. Life just does not happen that way.

4

My second mistake was lack of discipline. Third, lack of knowledge, and fourth poor habits. That formula equals zero results. I soon discovered that every time I experienced a setback, whether emotional or physical, I gave up and bounced right back to my old, comfortable destructive habits.

Another reason why I, along with millions of others, kept weight on was company parties. If you work, you know that company parties are all too frequent. Every time someone in my department celebrated a birthday, baby shower or job promotion, we had a party. And, of course, company parties are great temptations to over eat the wrong kinds of foods. Company parties and meetings are all too often catered with unhealthy types of foods and I found myself consuming too many potato chips, pretzels, pastries, nuts, cakes and soda. Also, as discussions heated in meetings, the more I ate. I guess you could say I was a compulsive eater. One of the hardest things I ever had to overcome was compulsive and emotional eating, but once I made a conscious effort, I successfully changed my routine and eliminated it forever. I noticed that if I had an urge to reach for a donut or cookies, I chose fruit or whole-wheat crackers instead; I felt physically better the remaining part of the day. After I got used to fruits and whole foods, I found that if I ate foods containing high amounts of refined sugar, they gave me a synthetic (strung out) high feeling. I then realized I should stick with the healthier choices.

My suggestion to you is, the next time you attend either a company party or social event, is to reach for the healthier food choices. If none are available, simply eat a minimum amount, then go out to a restaurant that serves healthy meals, or go home and prepare a quick healthy meal. I sometimes eat at home before attending a party if I know in advance what is being served is not healthy. The key is to only consume enough calories and fat that you know you will be able to burn off each day.

If you lead a busy lifestyle, sometimes cooking big meals just does not fit into your daily schedule. First and foremost, avoid fast food places that will defeat your purpose. There are approximately 30 grams of fat in just one burger, and if you also order fries and a soda, you will consume the maximum fat and calorie content for the entire day. And unless your lifestyle is extremely active, in order to burn off all your consumed fat and calories, it will convert to fat.

Now if you live alone and do not want to go home to an empty apartment or house, either invite a friend or go alone to a nice restaurant with a desirable atmosphere without screaming kids flying in every direction. Replace that burger with turkey, fish or chicken. Preferably find a restaurant with a healthy menu. Who knows, maybe one day you will meet someone special at that same restaurant and end up sharing an enjoyable, healthy meal together.

Develop a mind set for a gradual but permanent change. Think of it as a journey to your long hoped for dream—only this time your dream will become a reality. Be courageous and dare to live your dream.

If others ridicule you once you begin to lose weight and really look good, learn to shun them and understand they are not capable and willing to take a positive step to better themselves. Misery loves company, and chances are they are jealous of your accomplishments. People will love you when you are overweight and miserable like they are and will dislike you when you are thin and happy. Begin to live for yourself and leave others to their style of living choices.

Before you begin any new diet or exercise program, see your doctor and get a physical examination. A complete exam is best, including a blood workup. If you have high blood pressure, high levels of cholesterol, diabetes or any other health problems, your selection of foods may vary from the norm.

Chapter 3

DEVELOPING NEW HEALTHY HABITS

Change is an essential part of life, but many people are resistant to change. I cannot tell you how many times I tried to change my old bad habits to better ones—I have lost count.

It took about one year to find the successful formula to permanent weight loss, healthy eating and a healthier lifestyle.

The first step is what I refer to as "habit replacement." Begin by replacing one bad habit at a time. Then one week later, after you are comfortable with the first habit replacement, replace another bad habit with a new healthy one, and so on and so forth. Before you know it, in just a couple of months, you should have an entire set of new habits.

My first habit replacement was each morning I replaced drinking coffee with freshly juiced fruit from my juicer. The second habit replacement was from soda to 100% juice or skim milk with lunch. For dinner, I either drank water, skim milk or juice instead of soda. With those first simple habit replacements, I reduced my calorie intake as well as developed healthier habits.

One of my major habit replacements was the way I grocery shopped. I replaced all my processed foods like refined white flour, refined sugar, prepared foods, whole milk, and etc. with low-fat items and whole foods.

Examples of whole foods are a wide selection of fresh produce like fruits and vegetables, whole grain bread, whole grain flour, whole grain pancake mix, whole grain instant rice, honey instead of white sugar and the list goes on. I also cut down on eating red meats and replaced them with fresh fish like salmon, cod, haddock, tuna steaks, lamb, turkey meats, turkey bacon and stopped buying pork products. A ton of fat is in all pork products. I carefully read all food labels before I purchase them, cutting down on foods with additives and preservatives. I also avoid frozen foods that have been prepared with breaded or batter ingredients. I now buy crackers, cereals, cookies with low sodium and are low in fat. I replaced eating ice cream with frozen yogurt. A wide variety of frozen yogurt is available and is quite tasty. I eat it with fresh strawberries or berries.

The most difficult bad habit to break was snacking. Snacking in moderation is ok, but remember, it is *what* you eat that matters. I eat breakfast at 7:00 a.m., so around 9:30 a.m. or 10:00 a.m. I am hungry again. But, of course, it is too early to eat lunch, so I usually eat one banana or an apple with spring water. A low-fat granola bar or something similar will also satisfy your hunger until lunchtime. My afternoon snack is around 3:00 p.m. or 4:00 p.m., when I eat a handful of low sodium wheat thins, Triscuits or an apple.

My final habit replacement was additional exercises to my existing workout. I increased my workout by 30 minutes every Monday, Wednesday and Friday. Believe me, you have got to move it to lose it. Despite what some diets state, it is imperative to burn the calories you consume to prevent them from turning into fat. Fat is harder to burn than calories. If you have not exercised before, start out with an easy workout. Whether your workout is walking or aerobics, you will increase your metabolism by adding exercise to your schedule.

Since I have been working out for 15 years, the adjustment was not difficult to deal with as for those who are couch potatoes. If you have a more sedentary lifestyle, my suggestion is to start out slow and easy. Consult with your physician before starting a workout, especially if you suffer from heart disease or any other type of disease.

Since you cannot add more hours to a day, the only other alternative is to adjust your time to fit your schedule. One suggestion is to get up a half hour earlier every day. You would be amazed at how much more can be accomplished with just 30 extra minutes. Begin to use this time to read the morning paper, watch news on TV or even have time to eat breakfast at home as opposed to grabbing a fast meal at a fast food place or company cafeteria. Slowly, and only when you feel ready, start a morning workout routine like walking for a mile or so. As a warning, start slowly then after one week add ¼ mile so that eventually you are walking at least 3 miles each morning. You may end up walking a lot farther, but starting slowly is the key. Many people make the mistake of over doing their workout and they feel stiff and sore for the next few days, finally giving up their workout routine. If you gently introduce a new exercise routine into your schedule, the results will be lasting.

To help make our new lifestyle a permanent one, introduce your plan to your family. Replace foods that tempt you in your first steps of habit replacement. Remove all the unhealthy foods like potato chips, cookies, sodas, and candy and replace them with things like fresh apples, bananas, peaches, grapes, sugar-free cookies and candies. I am sure you will hear some whining and complaining from your husband and kids, but when they experience more energy, better concentration and even excess weight loss themselves, you will receive many praises and thanks for your efforts.

If you are successful in changing only a few bad habits, you are on you way to a healthier lifestyle and the rest will eventually fall into place.

The bottom line in habit replacement is to stop and think each and every time you reach out to grab for your usual grocery item or that donut. Think of the dramatic consequences you will suffer each time you consume a food product high in sugar, fat or sodium. Let your conscience be your guide and you will feel much better yourself—the complements will be ongoing as well.

Chapter 4

NEW GROCERY LIST

Grocery shopping for the right foods is one of the most essential keys to successful weight loss. Since each day brings new and sometimes stressful events into your life, it is imperative to have a well-stocked kitchen. It is suggested that you stock your kitchen and shop only once a week, or if you can afford it, shop every two weeks except for staples like milk, butter, bread, etc. Shopping every day is not only stressful and unnecessary, but also expensive.

A well-planned shopping trip will affect your selections as to the quality and quantity you buy. I have a home computer and keep a master grocery list that I edit weekly. I then simply print it out and go to town.

Reading labels is the only way to choosing safe food items. Some low-fat products contain high sodium and cholesterol contents, which defeats your goal. Also, some foods labeled with no cholesterol have a high content of fat, i.e. some granola bars can have high amounts of fat, sodium, sugar and cholesterol, again canceling out your purpose to consuming less calories and fat.

Reading labels and package information should be an important habit replacement effort. If you view your shopping as a fun adventure and not as a chore, it will become enjoyable. Grocery shopping became so enjoyable for me that I started a business shopping for other people. It is a win-win situation—I make money plus educate people about healthy shopping and eating habits.

Have you heard the cliché "never grocery shop when you are hungry?" Shopping for food on an empty stomach is dangerous to your health and your pocket book. If you plan to shop and are hungry, but do not have time to prepare something at home, take time to stop at a healthy place and grab a bite. You could even temporarily satisfy your appetite by eating fruit or crackers. That way you will avoid picking up fattening items or unnecessary snacks that you need to avoid.

Many prepackaged foods, frozen and low-cal meals are filled with sodium, creating water retention. Some low-calorie meals contain small food portions, leaving you starving in one or two hours. Portions too small are not the best method of eating.

The best starting point in your grocery store is the produce section. It is usually located at the front of the store, and then simply work your way up and down each food aisle. I write my grocery list according to how I walk the store.

Suggested Foods

Before you start the Undiet Diet, the following are suggested staples and food items to re-stock your kitchen. It is not necessary to replace everything in your kitchen in one shopping trip, but each week it is best to add a few items from this list so that eventually all the healthy staples are in your cupboard.

Recommended Foods	Foods to Avoid
Whole-wheat flour	white flour
Honey	refined sugar
Whole wheat bread	white bread
Whole-wheat pancake mix	buttermilk pancake mix
Whole-wheat pasta	
Whole-oat oatmeal	instant oatmeal
Butter (low-sodium)	margarine
Skim or 1% milk	whole milk
Non-fat yogurt	cream cheese
Frozen yogurt	ice cream
Sugar-free ice cream	
Fat-free cottage cheese	
Fat-free cheese	
Turkey bacon	pork bacon
Chicken (skinless)	pork products

Recommended Foods

Lean hamburger
Salmon
Cod fish
Any cold-water fish
Healthy Choice pasta sauce
Fat-free salad dressing

Pure maple syrup
Rice cakes
Whole-wheat crackers
Popcorn (low-fat, low sodium)
Oatmeal & raisin cookies
Fructose-made cookies
Fruit bars
Tofu
Veggie or soy burgers

Foods to Avoid

ground chuck
catfish
clams
crab
shrimp
eat small amounts
Of shellfish

Suggested Cooking Oils—Cold Pressed Only

Butter
Olive oil
Canola oil
Sunflower oil
Sesame oil
Soybean oil
Nut oil
Safflower oil
Corn oil

Foods to eat in moderation
Uric acid forming foods = 40%

ACID ASH

Starches and Sugars (20%)

Barley
Bran
Breads (whole wheat)
Cereals (all kinds)
Cornmeal
Crackers
Doughnuts
Dry beans
Dry peas
Flour (whole wheat)
Gravies (all kinds)
Hominy
Jelly (all kinds)
Macaroni
Noodles
Pancakes (whole wheat)
Potatoes
Preserves
Pudding (low-fat)
Rice (whole wheat, brown or wild)
Rye
Spaghetti
Sugar (all kinds—minimal)
Syrups (all kinds)
Tapioca

Protein (20%)

cashews
cheese
eggs
fish
hazelnuts
hickory nuts
hazelnuts
lentils
meats (no pork)
olives
peanuts
peanut butter
pine nuts
pistachio nuts
poultry
walnuts

ACID ASH—continued

Starches and Sugars (20%)   **Protein (20%)**

Waffles
**50% of Vegetables and Fruits
Should Be Eaten Raw (uncooked)**

CLEANSING FOODS (60%)

Vegetables   **Fruits**

Vegetables	Fruits
Artichokes	apples
Asparagus	apricots
Beans	avocado
Beets	bananas
Broccoli	berries
Brussels sprouts	cantaloupe
Cabbage	cherries
Carrots	citron
Cauliflower	currants
Celery	dates
Chard	figs
Cucumbers	grapefruit
Eggplant	grapes
Endive	lemons
Garlic	limes
Kale	melons
Lettuce (all kinds except iceberg)	nectarines

CLEANSING FOODS (60%)—Continued

Vegetables

Leaks
Mushrooms
Okra
Onions
Oyster plant
Parsley
Parsnips
Peas
Peppers
Pimentos
Potatoes (with skins)
Pumpkin
Radishes
Rhubarb
Rutabagas and Sauerkraut

Fruits

olives
oranges
papaya
passion fruit
peaches
persimmons
pineapple
plums
raisins
raspberries
quince
strawberries
tangerines

Chapter 5

GRADUAL WEIGHT LOSS

Gradual weight loss is safer than following a fast food diet. Avoid yo-yo dieting, which is consuming too little calories and starving your body. This will slow your metabolism resulting in slow weight loss. People who practice yo-yo dieting end up gaining more weight back plus more. It is very unhealthy and could be life threatening.

Remember, you may not see a difference in your actual weight at first because muscle weight is heavier than fat weight. It is a good idea to keep track of your inches by measuring yourself once a week. You want to lose at a slow rate to maintain good health. One of your objectives is to also boost your immune system to keep you from getting sick while losing weight. Too many people go on crash diets and lose weight too fast, subsequently lowering their immune system, subjecting themselves to viruses resulting in colds and infections. Be patient, weight loss will happen and it will stay off if you follow suggestions in this book.

Permanent weight loss involves changing many aspects of your lifestyle, including but not limited to your eating habits, attitude, exercise and any emotional difficulties you may have. All of these areas must be dealt with and managed to successfully lose weight and keep it off.

The first and main focus is improving your eating habits, as previously discussed in Chapter 3. Habit replacement is the major key factor in successfully changing the way you eat.

Another key factor is that you must begin some sort of exercise routine, like walking 30 minutes a day. It is best to start out by walking slowly for about 30 minutes three times a week. Once you are comfortable with walking three times a week, increase it by adding one more day until you are walking 30 minutes for 5 days. Walking will increase your energy level as well as your strength. Depending on how you feel, you may want to add free weights, aerobics, and swimming to your routine. Gradual increases in your exercise routine will burn off the fat. If you increase your exercises too fast, you will crash and burn. Exercise may increase your appetite so be careful *what* you eat after your workout. If you satisfy your appetite with foods high in fat or sugar content, you will defeat your purpose.

Counting calories is also an important factor in gradual weight loss, but before you begin counting, it is equally important to replace all the junk food you consume with fruits and vegetables and sugar-free items.

After you have accustomed yourself to a healthy way of eating, start keeping a food journal. Jot down each day's meals you consume (it is important to include every piece of food to be fair to yourself), and how you feel each day. If you are more stressed on a particular day, you may find yourself eating more.

Purchasing a juicer machine could be the wisest decision you will ever make. Be sure to thoroughly read the booklets included with your juicer, as it gives vital information from recipes to cleaning your fruits and vegetables. If you juice only once or twice a day, along with healthy eating and exercising, I guarantee you will see and feel inches melt away in as little as two to three weeks.

Your goal is also to determine how much food to eat at each meal and then only eat that much. As tempting as it is to stuff yourself during the holidays, parties and business meetings, simply turn away from the excess and leave overeating to the other people. Absolutely do not starve yourself though. I have encountered a few people who boast about how they skip breakfast and lunch, then make up for lost meals at dinner time. A warning to those who practice this method—you are playing Russian roulette with your health! Never, I repeat never skip meals.

Those who expect long-term results from indulging in periods of starvation are sadly mistaken. The only results that come from starvation are weight gain and eventually illness. Your body's metabolism will actually slow itself down and store fat.

Gradually reduce your food portion size. Together with an exercise routine, this should result in weight loss. Never try to lose any more than one or two pounds a week. If you lose too much too fast, you may lose muscle tissue as well.

It has been tested and proven that more meals a day can actually help you gradually lose weight and maintain a desired weight. Eating approximately six small-portioned meals a day seems to be the magic formula. Once you have successfully achieved eating smaller portions at regular mealtime, you can now start increasing meals. This is accomplished by taking in the same number of calories in six meals as three meals a day. The following is an example of how to stay in control of your hunger and which may prevent you from bingeing.

8:00 a.m.	Hot oatmeal with honey Toasted bagel Fresh juice from juicer
10:00 a.m.	Piece of fruit
12:00 p.m.	Turkey sandwich on whole-wheat bread Carrot sticks Sugar-free cookies or nonfat cake
2:30 p.m.	Bowl of soup Whole-wheat crackers Low-fat cheese Nonfat milk or water
5:30 p.m.	Pasta Tomato sauce Steamed or fresh vegetables Low-fat fruit dessert
7:30 p.m.	Frozen yogurt Fruit water

Make sure you drink plenty of water throughout each day. Six to eight 8-oz. glasses of water a day is recommended. Drinking water also helps wash toxins out of your body and speeds weight loss.

Your mind rules your body, so create a mindset and take that first step to successful long-term weight loss and practice what you read in this book. Again, please visit your doctor and get a complete physical exam before starting the Undiet Diet and exercise program.

Once you lose at least ten pounds, reward yourself—safely. Go out and buy yourself a new outfit or take a short trip to the beach or mountains. If it is wintertime, go skiing or ice-skating. If you continue to reward yourself at certain weight loss milestones, you will feel much better about yourself, physically and emotionally, therefore eventually maintaining your perfect weight. Remember, fad diets, pills and drinks that promise fast results only leave you with an empty feeling in the end that will only cause you additional weight gain in a week or so also causing you to slip back into your old bad habits and lifestyle.

Chapter 6

SATISFY CRAVINGS SAFELY

Habit replacement and gradual lifestyle changes do not have to include deprivation. If you completely cut out all of your favorite foods and deprive yourself of all treats, chances are you will wind up bingeing and falling back into your old habits, canceling out months of hard work.

If you understand the devastating effects that depriving yourself has on your health, then you are on the right path to permanent weight loss. Many people make the detrimental choice of deprivation in order to achieve quick results. This may produce a temporary change in weight, but its long-term effects are devastating. Some of the effects may be losing your balance, losing your ability to make sound decision, blackouts, lack of energy, and in extreme cases, cease to exist. These people also gain back every pound in a subconscious attempt to get back every ounce of satisfaction they missed from depriving themselves.

When you replace unhealthy habits with healthy ones, life will become freer from guilt as well as reducing your fat intake. An example is eating great tasting frozen yogurt to replace high-fat ice cream. Finding new ways to satisfy old appetites with nonfat foods will enable you to lose weight. You will experience more energy since your body will be running more efficiently.

Once you begin satisfying your cravings in a healthy way, you will also actually crave less food because you will be putting a higher quality of food in your body. Refer to Chapter 8, *Simple Meal Suggestions*, for juice recipes that will eliminate cravings for sugar, salt and sour foods.

Sometimes food cravings stem from habit, boredom, or emotional upset. You may not even be hungry and want something besides food, but food fills that void. Try to identify your real craving and satisfy it in a healthy way. For example, if you are craving something sweet, eat fruit. The natural fructose will satisfy your sweet tooth. Cravings are based more on habit rather than hunger. Therefore, replace your old habits with healthy ones. Another example of a craving is you may have a consistent mid-evening snack. Try exercising, like walking instead of eating. If you get your mind off the need for satisfying the unhealthy cravings, you will squash that craving. Occasionally, you may have an extremely strong craving for a particular food like chocolate. Go ahead and satisfy that craving, but only with small portions.

When you think about it, eating junk food for snacks or meals is abusing your body, and your body greatly suffers. In my opinion, poor nutrition results in illness and disease, and in extreme cases, even death. Take a look at third world countries with lack of food—children are dying every three minutes from diseases due to poor nutrition. We should consider ourselves very fortunate because in America we have a million food choices—it is very important to make the healthy ones.

Chapter 7

WEIGHT LOSS MANAGEMENT
MAINTAINING YOUR DESIRED WEIGHT

Anyone can lose weight, but the majority fails in keeping it off. That is where weight loss management and maintaining a desired weight come into play. If you follow these four steps, you will succeed in permanent weight loss.

Step 1:

Eliminate foods high in fat, such as bacon and processed meats, junk food, processed and prepared foods, gravy, rich sauces, ice cream and excessive amounts of nuts.

Replace fried foods that are high in fat, such as meat, with broiled, boiled or baked lean meat. Steam fresh vegetables instead of boiling them—or eat them raw. Try to eliminate buying canned or processed vegetables and fruits also add more legumes to your diet.

Try juicing fresh fruits and vegetables. There are many affordable juicers on the market today that include juicing recipes. I prefer to juice fruits because I don't eat them fast enough and they rot in my refrigerator.

Why should you juice fresh fruits and vegetables instead of buying bottled juice? First, it is absolutely fresh, which is important because nutrients lose a lot of value in as little as 30 minutes after juicing. Second, juice from a juicer is not pasteurized, which means cooked—it is filled with the living cells that are vital to good health.

Lastly, fresh juice is pure and free from additives and preservatives. Juices made fresh and consumed instantly contain 95% of the food value of a fruit or vegetable, releasing nourishment to your entire body through the bloodstream.

Remember the old saying, "eat live foods, be alive—eat dead foods, live dead." It is true—after I changed my diet to primarily include live foods, my energy level is higher from the time I rise in the morning until I fall asleep at night.

Step 2:

You have got to move it to lose it! Calories are the unit to measure the amount of energy in food. A certain amount of calorie intake is a must to retain an energy level. When you try to lose weight, you need to reduce the amount of calories to between 1200 and 1600 a day. One pound of body fat equals 3500 calories, therefore to lose weight, you will need to do some sort of exercise. Giving point values to foods and keeping scores or records of your meals do nothing to alleviate the cause of dietary imbalances and unhealthy lifestyle habits. When real-life circumstances that cause your old bad habits to arise and you go backwards without thinking, your self-esteem is knocked down.

It is imperative that you make a conscious effort to replace old destructive eating habits with healthy ones. It is better to start slowly with an exercise routine, whether it is walking, yoga, step aerobics or running. After one week, increase with an additional 10 minutes to your routine until you have reached what you consider a perfect workout.

Because muscle weighs more than fat, many people gain or maintain the same weight after toning and firming up a flabby body. However, after a couple of months, a regular exercise routine will generate a reduction of body fat and an increase of lean muscle.

Step 3:

Drink plenty of water. It is recommended that six to eight 8-oz. glasses of water each day be consumed. If you are living in a warmer climate, drink more. If your body becomes dehydrated, it will inhibit fat metabolism.

During your exercise workout, it may be best to carry a thermal water bottle with you so you can drink whenever you are thirsty.

Step 4:

Satisfy your cravings. Never deprive your body of calories when you are hungry. Depriving your body of food will make you want it more, creating bingeing and going off your successful path of permanent weight loss.

With healthy habit replacements, exercising and six small meals a day, you will prevent a rebound effect in the future.

It has been proven that 97% of people who choose crash diets, pills or diet drinks to lose weight fast, gain all their original weight back.

To achieve healthy permanent weight loss as part of your lifestyle, your eating and exercise habits must be realistic and enjoyable.

Chapter 8

SIMPLE MEAL SUGGESTIONS

The following are tasty, low-fat meal suggestions that are healthy and satisfying to you and your entire family.

These meals are interchangeable, so feel free to choose whatever meals your taste buds demand.

It is equally important to teach your children good eating habits since they learn from what they see and these are their crucial developmental years.

Eat vegetables raw or steamed to retain the fiber and vitamin benefits. Park your car far away from the door of your office or when you are shopping and use the stairs instead of the elevator. Plan a specific exercise around your schedule, or try to form an exercise group with your friends so the routine is fun. Learn to recognize your stress factors and reduce your stress in ways other than eating. Keep a positive attitude and self-image by concentrating on your current successes.

Sunday

Breakfast

Fresh plums
Sliced raw apple
Banana with chopped nuts
Whole grain bread
Beverage: skim milk or fresh juice

Lunch

Lettuce and tomato salad, diet dressing
Broiled chicken (4 oz.)
½ dish turnips (4-1/2 oz.)
Mushrooms (3 oz.)
Strawberries (3 oz.)
Beverage: skim milk, ice tea or fresh juice

Dinner

Scrambled eggs and asparagus (4 oz.)
(2 egg whites, 3 stalks of asparagus)
1 dish mixed greens (4 oz.)
1 apple (4 oz.)
Beverage: water or fresh juice

Monday

Breakfast

Oatmeal (not instant)
Juice or 1 whole orange
2 fresh pear halves
Beverge: coffee (no sugar) or fresh juice

Lunch

Tomato & lettuce salad with diet dressing
1 dish turnips
2/3-cup string beans
2 peach halves
Beverage: decaffeinated tea or fresh juice

Dinner

Lettuce & onion salad (4 oz.) with diet dressing
(1/2 cup lettuce, 4 small onions)
4 oz. lean meat (veal, chicken, turkey, beef or lamb)
6 asparagus stalks with dressing
2/3-cup pineapple
Beverage: ice tea or fresh juice

<u>Tuesday</u>

Breakfast

Whole grain muffin or bagel with butter (no margarine)
Dish of orange slices and raspberries
Beverage: skim milk or fresh juice

Lunch

Cabbage and pimento salad (7 oz.)
(1 cup cabbage, 2 slices pimento, 1 tbs. parsley)
1 hard-boiled egg (1-1/2 oz.)
1 dish carrots (2-1/2 oz.)
4 apricot halves (2-1/2 oz.)
Beverage: iced tea or fresh juice

Dinner

Shredded radish salad (6 oz.)
Codfish filet (4 oz.)
2/3-cup spinach (5 oz.)
1 cup squash (6 oz.)
¾ cup strawberries (3 oz.)
Beverage: iced tea, fresh juice or water

Wednesday

Breakfast

2 boiled eggs
Whole-wheat toast with butter
Dish of back or red currants with milk
Beverage: Coffee, tea or fresh juice

Lunch

Cucumber salad (6 oz.)
(1 large cucumber, 1 oz. shredded cabbage, lettuce, diet dressing)
Cottage cheese and chives (3 oz.)
Applesauce without sugar (4 oz.)
Beverage: fresh juice

Dinner

Vegetable salad with diet dressing (4 oz.)
1 dish boiled onions
Portion of lean meat or cottage cheese (4 oz.)
2/3-cup string beans
½ dish berries (any kind)
Beverage: water or fresh juice

Thursday

Breakfast

Wholegrain cereal with skim milk and honey
Dish fresh fruit
Beverge: skim milk or fresh juice

Lunch

Tomato stuffed with tuna
1 dish beets (4 oz.)
Red cabbage (2 oz.)
½ grapefruit
Beverage: iced tea or fresh juice

Dinner

Shredded cabbage salad (2 oz.)
1 small dish broccoli (3 oz.)
1 dish sauerkraut (4 oz.)
Lean round broiled steak (4 oz.)
1 dish prunes or cherries (3 oz.)
Beverage: fresh juice or water

Friday

Breakfast

Large dish of soft fruit (all kinds) with lemon, honey and skim milk
Beverage: coffee (no sugar) or fresh juice

Lunch

Asparagus salad (3 oz.)
(4 stalks asparagus, 1 leaf romaine lettuce, 1 onion, diet dressing)
Baked Cauliflower (4 oz.)
Young peas (4 oz.)
Carrots (3 oz.)
½ grapefruit
Beverage: fresh juice or iced tea

Dinner

Tomato stuffed with lettuce and diet dressing
Dish turnips (4-1/2 oz.)
Dish red cabbage (3 oz.)
Filet of broiled Haddock (4 oz.)
Dish of pears (1-1/2 oz.)
Beverage: fresh juice or water

Saturday

Breakfast

2 poached eggs
1 slice of whole-wheat bread with butter
½ grapefruit
Beverage: skim milk or fresh juice

Lunch

Celery and apple salad
(1 leaf romaine or red leaf lettuce, ½ apple)
1 dish of mixed beets and lettuce leaves (6 oz.)
1 cup sautéed mushrooms (6 oz.)
1 cup peaches (6 oz.)
Beverage: fresh juice or iced tea

Dinner

Shredded turnip salad
(1/2 cup turnips, leaf lettuce, diet dressing)
Peppers and tomatoes (6 oz.)
Roast beef (4 oz.)
2/3-cup pineapple (4 oz.)
Beverage: fresh juice or water

If you find yourself craving snacks in-between meals, try one of these healthy selections. Remember, everything in moderation!

SNACK IDEAS

Low sodium popcorn
Grapefruit
Strawberries
Berries (all kinds)
Grapes (green or red)
Peach
Pear
Apple
Banana
Wheat thins
Triscuits
Rice cakes
Low-fat mini pizzas
Carrot sticks
Frozen yogurt
Sugar-free yogurt
Herbal teas: green or black teas (decaffeinated)

FRESH JUICE IDEAS

Try one of the following juices each morning with your breakfast. These recipes are also excellent for mid-morning snacks instead of food.

Breakfast Drinks

Pineapple/Grapefruit Drink

1-1/2 grapefruit (peeled)
2 rings of pineapple

Pineapple/Orange Drink

2 rings of pineapple
2 peeled oranges

Pineapple/Strawberry Drink

3 rings of pineapple
8 strawberries

Pineapple/Strawberry/Apple Drink

1 Red Delicious apple
2 rings of pineapple
6 strawberries

Morning-Sunrise Cocktail

½ pink pineapple (peeled)
1 medium orange (peeled)
1 cup strawberries

Peach Delight

1 peach
1 orange (peeled)
Add chilled ½ cup sparkling mineral water

Creamsicle Drink

1 cup fresh-juiced oranges
½ cup fresh-juiced apples
1 tsp honey
¼ tsp vanilla extract
2 tbs nonfat dry milk or skim milk
2 ice cubes
Mix all ingredients in a blender on high until ice is liquefied. Drink immediately.

Strawberry Shake

½ cup sliced strawberries
¾ cup apple and orange juice
¼ cup nonfat dry milk or skim milk
4 ice cubes
Put strawberries into blender and liquefy. Add remaining ingredients and whip until mixture is thick and light. Pour into glasses and eat with spoon.

<u>Lunch Drinks</u>

Tomato Cocktail

Juice 3 large ripe tomatoes
(or 4-5 small tomatoes)
½ cucumber
1 stalk celery
Small slice lime (with peel)

Garden Special

Handful of spinach
5 or 6 carrots

Stress Reliever

4-5 carrots
½ apple (remove seeds)
¼ inch slice fresh ginger

Cantaloupe Shake

½ cantaloupe (with skin)
¼-inch ginger root

Luncheon Special

1 garlic clove
Small handful of spinach
4-5 carrots (remove greens)
2 stalks celery
Parsley for garnish

Heartburn Reliever

¼ head cabbage
1 stalk celery
2 carrots (remove greens)

<u>Dinner Drinks</u>

Immune Booster

4 carrots
3 sprigs parsley
2 stalks celery
2 garlic cloves

Liver Energizer

3 carrots
½ beet

Calcium Cocktail

3 kale leaves
Small handful parsley
4-5 carrots (remove greens)
½ apple (remove seeds)

Liquid Veggie Garden Drink

Handful parsley
3 beet tops
2 stalks celery
4 carrots (remove greens)

Pancreas Tonic

3 romaine lettuce leaves
4-5 carrots (remove greens)
Handful of green beans
2 Brussels sprouts

Eye Opener

2 endive leaves
Handful parsley
4-5 carrots (remove greens)
2 stalks celery

Ultimate Garden Delight

3 broccoli flowerets
1 garlic clove
4-5 carrots or 2 tomatoes
2 stalks celery
½ green pepper

Cleansing Tonic

¼-inch slice ginger root
1 beet
½ apple (remove seeds)
4 carrots (remove greens)

Cravings

Dealing with food cravings means getting to the root of the cause for particular food urges. Even though your body is telling to eat a whole quart of chocolate ice cream or an entire bag of pretzels, that is not what your body needs. Chances are it needs something completely different. Identify what you crave and put into practice drinking the following juice drinks to satisfy those cravings. If a particular drink is not listed in this book, research other books for drinks or foods to deal with unhealthy cravings.

The following are drinks to satisfy and suppress cravings for sweets and chocolates, salty foods, peanut butter and even sour foods.

Sugar Cravings

Ginger Hopper

¼-inch slice ginger root
4-5 carrots (remove greens)
½ apple (remove seeds)

Cleansing Tonic

¼-inch slice ginger root
1 beet
½ apple (remove seeds)
4 carrots (remove greens)

45

Mineral Tonic

Handful of parsley
2 turnip leaves
1 kale leaf
4-5 carrots (remove greens)

<u>Salt Cravings</u>

Potassium Broth

Handful of parsley
Handful of spinach
4-5 carrots (remove greens)
2 stalks celery

Garlic Cooler

Handful of parsley
1 garlic clove
4-5 carrots (remove greens)
2 stalks of celery

Tomato Drink

Handful of spinach
Handful of parsley
2 tomatoes
½ green pepper
Dash of Tabasco sauce

Peanut Butter Cravings

Ginger Hopper

¼-inch slice ginger root
4-5 carrots (remove greens)
½ apple (remove seeds)

Pineapple Cooler

3-inch slice pineapple (with skin)
½ apple (remove seeds)
½ cup coconut milk

Garlic Cooler

Handful of parsley
1 garlic clove
4-5 carrots (remove greens)
2 stalks of celery

Sour Food Cravings

Calcium-Rich Drink

3 kale leaves
Small handful of parsley
4-5 carrots (remove greens)
½ apple (remove seeds)

Ann's Delicious Lemonade

3-4 apples (remove seeds)
¼ lemon (with peel)

Chlorophyll Delight

3 beet tops
Handful of parsley
Handful of spinach
4 carrots (remove greens)
½ apple (remove seeds)

Chapter 9

EATING OUT

If your life is active and very busy, cooking at home every day is not always possible. Sooner or later you are going to be forced to eat out and your choices of landing at a fast-food place will be high. Remember to make a conscious effort to think before you pull into the driveway of an unhealthy place. However, many fast food places have added healthier meals to their menu. You could order a baked potato with a side salad. Instead of using their salad dressing, carry your own fat-free dressing to add to their salad. Also, some fast food restaurants charbroil their foods therefore you can enjoy a tasty skinless chicken with a salad topped with your own dressing and lemonade or diet drink.

If you prefer a fine dining restaurant, try to find out their menu before you sit down to order. One time I went to a very nice restaurant in my area that I thought offered a wide variety of foods and wanted to eat fresh broiled fish with whole grain rice. When the waiter approached me to take my order, I asked if they could broil or poach the fish. He responded stiffly, "no." He said they only fried their breaded fish.

I asked him to check with the chef if he would make an exception. After all, the customer is always right. He again responded, "No, we don't do that here." I calmly got up out of my chair and told him, "good evening" and walked out of the restaurant. I found a restaurant around the corner that was willing to poach the fish I ordered.

You do not have to compromise your diet simply because a particular restaurant does not serve healthy food. You are in control of your diet and there are many restaurants in your town or city that will serve healthier meals.

Many cities have a few specialty health food restaurants that offer such menus as vegetarian meals, turkey lasagna, low-fat Mexican meals, oven-roasted chicken dinners, fresh broiled fish dishes and much more.

Most restaurants offer full salad bars. Foods to avoid are excessive cheese, pasta items, eggs with yolks, bacon bits and diced meat. All these foods have high fat, and high calorie count. Unless you plan to do a high-powered workout for one to two hours a day, I suggest you limit these high fat foods. To top your salad, olive oil and vinegar or diet dressing are excellent choices, or you could carry your favorite diet dressing with you.

Changing the way you eat can be a very enjoyable and satisfying adventure. Bon Appetite!

Chapter 10

WHEN THINGS GET TOUGH

To simply read this book will not produce results for any weight loss, whether it is temporary or permanent. You must practice what you read. I will be the first to admit that changing habits is not an easy feat. There will be many temptations to quit, even in the beginning of your weight loss management. It will take more than will power to lose weight. You may even reach your goal, lose all your desired weight, and then fall back in to all your original bad habits, erasing your efforts.

This is where faith enters the picture. Have you ever noticed that those who have a strong belief in God seem to heal faster and are more content and happy? It is true.

Approximately eight years ago, I lost my best friend, my mother. I also had just given birth to my first child, was in a bad marriage and the stress of my job was killing me. One evening while watching TV, just as I was about to change the channel, a religious program came on. My attention was drawn to the pastor as he spoke of sick and troubled people. He seemed to be addressing my exact problems. At the end of the 30-minute program he suggested reading one verse from any chosen book in the Bible every day. He stated that by reading the Bible each day, the quality of life would dramatically improve. I thought what do I have to lose and started that night. I not only read one verse, but also read the entire book of John. The following night I read one verse from the book of Mark. I continued this routine, and to this day, have not stopped. When everyone is asleep, in the quiet of my bedroom, I continue to read a verse every night before I go to bed. After starting the readings and after only one month, I noticed a change in my life. My life slowly turned around for the better. I then started going back to church. Exactly three years later, I made a decision to move to another state and subsequently met my husband. Bad times made a mysterious turn for the better. And now when logic tells me a situation will turn out one way, it takes an unexpected turn toward a positive outcome. And I know exactly who is alive and with me at all times—God.

If you listen carefully, you will hear God speaking and guiding you through your life. That idea you have, an intuitive feeling, or even some sort of sign given to you may be God speaking to you. He speaks to everyone in a unique manner.

Proverbs 16:1-3:

> The plans of the mind belong to man,
> But the answer of the tongue is from the Lord.

> All the ways of a man are pure in his own
> Eyes, but the Lord weighs the spirit.

> Commit your work to the Lord,
> And your plans will be established.

Chapter 11

SUCCESS AT LAST

Several people sent me their success stories, thanking me for an easy, realistic way to lose weight permanently. One story in particular impressed me so much that I asked her permission to put her story in my book.

An environmental engineer was obese two years ago. She carried more than 300 pounds on her 5-foot, 2-inch body. Today she is maintaining a weight of 120 pounds.

She came to understand the importance of reading food labels and monitoring her food intake together with walking and stretching exercises.

"For many years I didn't care what I poured into my body," she wrote. "Now I do."

"I learned that label information can play an important role in weight management."

In the past, diet-conscious people could not always count on the food labels to give complete nutritional information. The information was required only when a food contained added nutrients or when nutrition claims appeared on the label. That has changed as a result of the Nutrition Labeling and Education Act of 1990, and regulations from the Food and Drug Administration and the U.S. Department of Agriculture.

Nutrition information is now bigger and in more readable type for almost all packaged foods. The information will also be near many fresh foods, like fruits and vegetables. On packaged foods, it will usually appear on the side on back of the package under the heading, "Nutrition Facts."

Remember, fat—not calorie content is the most important information for weight loss management on the food label. Fat is the densest source of calories, with 9 calories per gram, while carbohydrates and protein each have 4 calories per gram. Alcohol, although not a nutrient, provides 7 calories per gram. By limiting fat alone, you will likely lower your calories, and thereby reducing weight.

In the past, diet conscious people were told to focus entirely on calories, but the new trend is for them to monitor and reduce grams of fat.

It is advised to limit fat consumption to no more than 30 percent of your total day's calories. For example, most people who eat 2,000 calories a day should strive to limit their calories from fat to no more than 600 (2,000 x 0.30 = 600) or no more than 65 grams fat (600 calories divided by 9 calories per gram fat = 67, rounded to 65).

Whatever your calorie intake, you can still use the % Daily Values to get a general idea of how high or low a food is in the major nutrients. Of course, it is recommended to see a doctor, dietitian or nutritionist before you begin changing your diet, especially if you suffer from diabetes, heart disease or any other illnesses. These professionals can assist you to determine appropriate calories and fat levels that will allow healthy weight loss and still receive adequate nutrition. Your doctor or nutritionist will know if any drugs you are currently taking will inhibit certain food, vitamin and mineral absorption.

Check and double-check labels for food fiber. Fiber can be an important aid in weight maintenance because eating enough of it can help make you feel full, thus curbing your appetite.

Food and Drug Administration and the U.S. Department of Agriculture reference amounts are set at 11.5 grams of fiber per 1,000 calories, thus the Daily Value for fiber is 25 grams. This Daily Value is based partly on the National Cancer Institute's recommendation that Americans eat 20 to 30 grams fiber a day. For most people a fiber intake of at least 25 grams a day—100% of the Daily Value is desirable. Begin your search for fat, fiber and calorie information on the front of the food package. This is where food manufacturers often place statements about the nutritional benefits of their products. Some of these, i.e., "fat-free," "low-calorie," and "high-fiber" will be important information.

Beware though, when choosing foods that are labeled "fat-free" and "low-fat" because some of these foods, like low-fat cakes and cookies still may be high in calories due to added sugars. Always check the Nutrition Facts panel to get complete information.

The column headed "% Daily Value" is the place to start under "Nutrition Facts." The numbers in this column can quickly tell if a food is high or low in the nutrients listed. The % Daily Values for fat and fiber are especially important. If they are 5 or less, the food is considered low in that nutrient. Your goal should be to select, as much as possible, foods that have a % Daily Value for fat of 5 or less, and 5 and higher for fiber.

Your ultimate goal should be to select foods that together add up to about 100% of the Daily Value for each nutrient. You can occasionally select a higher fat item, like a slice of pound cake that provides about 15% of the Daily Value for fat, but monitor your other foods you eat that day and try not to go over 100% of the Daily Value for fat.

The idea is to give yourself enough flexibility in making food choices to keep your meals interesting, yet restricting the total daily fat intake and increase your total daily fiber intake.

I realize all this information may be overwhelming at first, so take your time and review all the information in this book until you have a good understanding of how to plan your meals, shop for healthy foods, read labels, and decide how and when you will begin your exercise routine. You are now on your way to a healthy way to permanent weight loss. Now you know why I entitled the book, "The Undiet Diet." There is no need to ever take another diet pill, consume unpleasant tasting diet drinks, and partake in grueling exercises ever again to lose weight. It is as simple as habit replacement. Simply replace your old habits with new ones, one habit at a time, so you don't overwhelm yourself.

It is now time to put these pages into action. I learned a long time ago that hands-on or actually doing something is the only way to see successful results! You will feel better and look better.